Finding JOY

On the Path of Divine Health and Wholeness

Joy Marlena Lambe

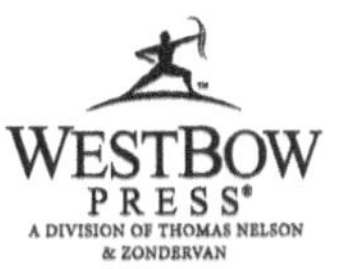

WESTBOW
PRESS®
A DIVISION OF THOMAS NELSON
& ZONDERVAN

WestBow Press books may be ordered through booksellers or by contacting:

WestBow Press
A Division of Thomas Nelson & Zondervan
1663 Liberty Drive
Bloomington, IN 47403
www.westbowpress.com
1 (866) 928-1240

Edited by John Anthony Rogers

ISBN: 978-1-9736-8751-1 (sc)
ISBN: 978-1-9736-8750-4 (hc)
ISBN: 978-1-9736-8752-8 (e)

Library of Congress Control Number: 2020903942

Print information available on the last page.

WestBow Press rev. date: 4/2/2020

With Appreciation

For all who walked alongside Joy, offering
encouragement and strength in times of weakness,
care and comfort in the presence of great pain,
reassurance in places of discouragement,
reminding of divine grace enfolding and sustaining

Contents

Foreword

SHE WAS THREE and I was seven when I first met Joy Marlena Lambe. I remember introducing myself to her and telling her that I liked her cute, white socks. I am sure she thought I was crazy. Four years is a big gap when you are so young; so our friendship did not really solidify until our teen years, when we spent summers writing, practicing and singing gospel songs in a group.

Joy was a gifted musician and writer, and she had a unique style, very different from what we called "church music" in those days. Even in her youth, her music communicated both questions and hope at the same time. I find myself smiling, crying and reflecting on that same depth of soul as I read and reread her journal.

For the past fifty years, I have observed many followers of Jesus Christ receive healing from physical disease and pain. Their victories have varied in scope and time: an unexplainable miraculous healing during prayer or Bible study; a gradual recovery while being treated by a medical specialist; a transition from their suffering that ushered them into heaven. Each journey was both personal and unique. But in most cases, the intense pain and suffering produced an intimacy with the healer, Jesus, that few have been able to share in words that others could benefit from.

This was not the case with my dear friend Joy Marlena Lambe. She chronicled her journey in words, examples and images that breathe God's kind of life into the reader. Her words help us understand that God's life goes beyond the physical and informs every ounce of our being. Her words remind us that when we are searching for one type of solution, such as physical healing, we are often surprised by healing that also rebalances our emotional, mental and spiritual self.

Her words help us to find Joy!

Dr. Chyanna Mull-Anthony
Pastor, International Gospel Center
Vice-President, Osborn Ministries International

Introduction

JOY MARLENA LAMBE learned that cancer cells were residing inside her in 2002. Twelve years later, in the spring of 2014, she wrote a letter to encourage a fellow traveler living with cancer:

> I was diagnosed in 2002 with a rare cancer called thymoma. It was and still is inoperable. I have been through years of chemo and radiation. I actually just finished my third time around with radiation about six weeks ago (second time within a year.)
>
> I have recognized and admit that over the years, my reliance has been greatly on the doctors and what they had to offer. Yes, I am a Christian, pray and believe, but in the back of my mind I was always waiting for that "wonder drug" from the doctors and it was always a big letdown when the new chemo didn't work.
>
> I have been treated with every chemotherapy possible and have exhausted all chemo avenues. There is no more that the doctors can do for me. I go and they monitor me, but that is the extent of it. All roads with them lead to a "Dead End" (pun intended). But don't get me wrong, doctors are extremely important. God made them for a reason and their knowledge has brought me through some really crucial and trying times.
>
> But the point still remains that God made them; so as Creator, He is greater than His creation. His ways, thoughts, knowledge and timing are on a

whole different level than we could ever begin to comprehend. And because of this fact, this is not the "end" of my story, only the beginning!

In March of 2015, Joy began a conversation with Freeda Bowers' book *Give Me 40 Days for Healing* (Bridge-Logos, 2007). Part of that conversation was journaling in response to Bowers' reflections on healing. Joy journaled on forty days from early March through mid-May.

On Thursday, February 18, 2016, Joy wrote this meditation in the same journal she had used in 2015:

> *My Intent. To Align my Being with Your Spirit, O Lord, so that when the Portal to Divine Health and Wholeness opens, I will by faith walk through. And as I do, I will be made whole. And on reaching the other side, infused with Your Healing Power, I will be ready to fulfill the Purpose for which You created me, my Destiny that You preordained for me before the world began.*

On the afternoon of Thursday, May 3, 2018, during her fifty-fourth trip around the sun, Joy's journey with cancer came to an end as she departed to her eternal home.

What follows are forty entries from Joy's 2015 journal on her journey toward what she refers to as Divine Health and Wholeness. The original entries were handwritten in a spiral-bound notebook. During the first six months of 2016, Joy transcribed a section labeled *Thoughts* from each of the first twenty-seven entries by reading them into a computer and then editing them as they appear here. She did not transcribe the final thirteen entries, days twenty-eight through forty, which were transcribed later for this book.

Wounds inflicted, grace imparted; tethered to fear, released by truth and love; conformity and creativity; individuality and community; uncertainty and faith; regret and gratitude; constraint and freedom. Joy Marlena Lambe, in her journey with cancer, and in her quest for healing and meaning, for divine health and wholeness, experienced these deep currents of the spiritual life as she embraced the divine treasure in her vessel of clay (2 Corinthians 4:7). The intimate entries from her journal that comprise *Finding Joy* manifest her emergent abiding with Christ, who gave her much hope and strength, much courage and love. Though faced with seemingly insurmountable adversity, she experienced the promise that in all circumstances, divine grace is at work effecting the divine will in and through those who love God and are learning to live and love in accord with God's plan (Romans 8:28).

John Anthony Rogers, Editor

The Journal

1

It's a Finished Work

March 5, 2015 (Thursday)

1 PETER 2:24 — *Who Himself bore our sins in His own body on the tree, that we, having died to sins, might live for righteousness—by whose stripes you were healed.*

PSALM 107:20 — *He sent His word and healed them, / And delivered them from their destructions.*

✝✝✝

Thanking God for this day/opportunity.

Sang: "Speak to My Heart, Lord"
　　　"I Am Well, I Am Whole"

Quoted Healing Scriptures:

> Psalm 103:2 – Bless the Lord, O my soul, And forget not all His benefits.

> Proverbs 9:10-11 – The fear the Lord is the beginning of wisdom... For by me, days multiplied, years added.

> 1 John 4:4 – Greater is He that is within me.

> Isaiah 54:17 – No weapon formed against me shall prosper.

Mark 7:27 – Healing is the children's bread; Romans 8:27 – I am an heir and joint-heir.

Psalm 118:17 – I will not die, but live and proclaim Your works.

Psalm 107:20 – He sent His Word and healed them, and delivered them from their destruction.

1 Peter 2:24 – By His stripes I am/I was healed.

Proverbs 3:5, 7-8 – Trust in the Lord with all thine heart… Be not wise in your own eyes… Health… Strength.

Isaiah 40:31 – They that wait on the Lord shall renew their strength. They shall mount up on wings like eagles. They shall run and not get weary. They shall walk and not faint.

Isaiah 55:11 – So shall My Word be that goes forth from My mouth. It shall not return to Me void, but it shall accomplish what I please, and it shall prosper in the thing for which I sent it.

Isaiah 58:8 – Then your light shall break forth like the morning, your healing shall spring forth speedily, and your righteousness shall go before you, the glory of the Lord shall be your rear guard.

Jeremiah 33:6 – Behold I will bring health and healing, I will heal them and reveal to them the abundance of peace and truth.

I woke up very nauseous; but after praying, singing and quoting Scripture, the nausea passed! All praise, honor and glory to God! Thank you, Lord!

It was a good day! No nausea returned. Still bigger battles to fight. More focus and quietness needed on my part. I have pinpointed four individuals to pray for during this journey. I sent out my first entry to them and gifted them with the digital version of Bowers' book. I look forward to their progress and mine. Thank you, Lord, for a wonderful day!

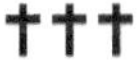

I am "healed under attack…. 'I am already healed, and I refuse to settle for anything less than a full manifestation of that healing'" (Bowers, 72).

✝✝✝

2

Save Me, Lord

March 6, 2015 (Friday)

Jeremiah 17:14 — *Heal me, O Lord, and I shall be healed; / Save me, and I shall be saved, / For You are my praise.*

✝✝✝

It has been another amazing day! Today I found myself singing "I Surrender All." That was a song that I played and sang back in the day. I prayed to God, telling Him that I surrender. It was in my spirit, and I meant it from my heart.

I was taken aback when I read the devotional today, "Save Me, Lord," which talked about accepting Jesus Christ as Saviour and Lord as a prerequisite for healing. Though I don't agree with that being true in all cases, the issue for me was that it is easy to accept Jesus as Saviour but difficult to accept Him as, or allow Him to be, Lord.

Perhaps it is the nature of the physical man, or perhaps it is the touch of eternity within, that makes us feel invincible. Whatever it is, we think we can make it on our own, we know what's best for our lives, we have it all together, we can handle it, we don't need a Lord. And sometimes we think we barely need a Saviour.

But the truth is, we do. We can't even move without God saying so, and we definitely cannot save our own soul. We need a Saviour. And to make it in this world, to navigate our lives, we need a Leader, a Guide, a King, a Lord.

The problem is that we think with the devil's mentality: God is no more than a slave driver, an uncompassionate lord that only wants to lord over us, a dictator that suppresses and impoverishes his people. Sounds like the accuser himself, not God.

But God is love, and out of love He stepped down to earth. The Creator birthed through the creation gave us His very best, His all. He became as you and I are to understand our plight. The King became the Servant to teach us the way of love. (God spoke that in my heart today.) Who's the greatest? He signed our adoption papers in His own blood. He made us heirs and joint-heirs and calls us friend.

Our Creator, Protector, Champion, Deliverer, Healer, Saviour, Brother, Friend, and yes, my Lord…to You, I Surrender All!

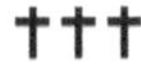

3
Choose Life
March 7, 2015 (Saturday)

DEUTERONOMY 30:19-20 — *I call heaven and earth as witnesses today against you, that I have set before you life and death, blessing and cursing; therefore choose life, that both you and your descendants may live; that you may love the* LORD *your God, that you may obey His voice, and that you may cling to Him, for He is your life and the length of your days.*

✝✝✝

Before I say anything…I Choose Life! There's a small billboard in front of the Catholic church that says, "Choose Life." It is an anti-abortion ad, but I had adopted it a long time ago as a decree for my healing. And here we are on day three: "Choose Life."

I am learning quickly that just saying it doesn't make it so. I can intellectualize it and comprehend its meaning, but there must be a transfer from my head to my heart, my spirit. But how?

That seed of life and healing in my brain must be watered by drops of faith. "Faith cometh by hearing, and hearing by the Word of God" (Romans 10:17). A constant deluge of the Word, total trust in the Son, and a weeding out of doubt and fear will produce deep roots that will infiltrate my whole being and finally take root, take hold in my heart, my spirit. Then the same Spirit that raised Jesus from the dead, which lives inside of me, will quicken my mortal body (Romans 8:11), and I will be whole! I will "be like a tree planted by the rivers of water" (Psalm 1:3).

I understand….Let the Son and the "rain" come now!

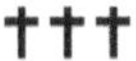

I found Freeda Bowers on YouTube. The entire "Give Me 40 Days for Healing" series is there. What a blessing! A free course with the author and her guest each day giving new insights and revelations as they journey with me for the forty days. God is showing out! LoL!

††† †

4

Keep God's Word in Your Heart

March 8, 2015 (Sunday)

PROVERBS 4:20-22 — *My son, give attention to my words; / Incline your ear to my sayings. / Do not let them depart from your eyes; / Keep them in the midst of your heart; / For they are life to those who find them, / And health to all their flesh.*

✝✝✝

Since day three, songs of Healing, Victory and Thanksgiving have been downloaded to my spirit from Heaven. It was so immediate. The melodies and words so distinctive. I went directly to my voice recorder and sang the lyrics. Last night I worked on some chords for one.

Some years ago, I was told twice, a confirmation, that my healing would come through my music. The songs would be for others but also for me.

I am offshore and I can't swim. I can't wade in and out anymore. I am way too deep. Only one lifeline: God's Word. Only one compass: The Holy Spirit. Only one destination: Wholeness. Only one anchor: The Lord.

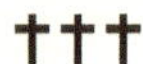

5

Forget Not All His Benefits

March 9, 2015 (Monday)

PSALM 103:1-3 — *Bless the Lord, O my soul; / And all that is within me, bless His holy name! / Bless the Lord, O my soul, / And forget not all His benefits: / Who forgives all your iniquities, / Who heals all your diseases.*

✝✝✝

Early this morning, the Lord led me to play and sing "Sweet Hour of Prayer." I can't tell you the last time I sang that song, but it was in my spirit, placed there by God; so I sang and played it. I knew the first verse, but I didn't know any others. So this afternoon I got the *Yes, Lord!* hymnal and looked it up. There are two verses. Verse two was confirmation to me.

Yesterday the lesson was about spending time with the Word for our healing to be manifested and God's desire to spend time with us One-on-one. And then out of the blue, these words:

> Sweet hour of prayer, sweet hour of prayer,
> Thy wings shall my petitions bear
> To Him whose truth and faithfulness
> Engage the waiting soul to bless.
> And since He bids me seek His face,
> Believe His Word and trust His grace,
> I'll cast on Him my every care
> And wait for thee, sweet hour of prayer.

How powerful! It was like He was talking to me through this verse, confirming all that has been said about cultivating an intimate relationship with Him. Then there are the scriptures about waiting and healing and renewed strength like the eagle.

Psalm 27:6 states, "I will sing and make music to the Lord." These are some lyrics I wrote today:

> As I wait…
> I will seek more of Your face.
> I will seek more of Your love.
> I will seek more of Your wisdom.
> I will seek more of Your peace.
> I will seek more of Your joy.
> I will seek more of Your strength.
> I will seek more of Your courage.
> I will seek more of Your patience.
> I will seek the more of You.

Pastor Freeda said this would happen: God meeting you when you take the time and He pouring out to you from His Word to the point where a separate Bible study must be established. Thank you, Lord, for meeting me again! I wait in faith—belief and intense expectation—for what God has in store.

More scriptures:

> Isaiah 40:21-31 (v. 31) — Those who wait on
> the Lord shall renew their strength. They shall
> mount up with *wings like eagles*. They shall run
> and not be weary; they shall walk and not faint.

Psalm 103:5 — Who satisfies your mouth with good things, so that *your youth is renewed like the eagles.*

Psalm 27:1-14 (v. 14) — Wait on the Lord: be of good courage, and He shall strengthen thine heart: wait, I say, on the Lord.

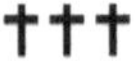

6

Break Agreement with Sickness

March 11, 2015 (Wednesday)

Amos 3:3 — *Can two walk together, unless they are agreed?*

✝✝✝

Much to process, and much to gain. For the first time, I came to terms with my words and fully understood how I have allowed them to negatively impact my health. Negative agreements with the dark side, whether conscious or unconscious, have hindered my progress towards wholeness.

One statement I often make is, "I'm hanging in there." And every time my dad says to me, "Abide." I really didn't get it until today. My words give acceptance to the symptoms. My dad's response gives no power to them and increases my faith by the power of God's Word. This response reaffirms my faith in the absolute truth of His Word and enables my spirit to realign itself with the Holy Spirit, who resides within to create the internal harmony and agreement needed to break all other agreements that are contrary to the Word of God. When I abide in His Word, I will know the truth, and it will set me free (John 8:31-32). When I abide in Him and in His Word, nothing will be withheld from me that I ask for.

So I ask, Holy Spirit, rise up within me, quicken my mortal body, and please manifest Your wholeness in me. Thank You for hearing and answering according to Your Word.

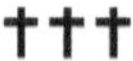

7
Appropriate Your Healing
March 12, 2015 (Thursday)

MATTHEW 9:28-29 — *And when He had come into the house, the blind men came to Him. And Jesus said to them, "Do you believe that I am able to do this?" They said to Him, "Yes, Lord." Then He touched their eyes, saying, "According to your faith let it be to you."*

✝ ✝ ✝

My words…
"Well, we're either going to believe this thing or we're not!"

Their words…
"Don't put all your eggs in one basket."
"It's a 50/50 chance."
"It's a toss-up."
"Don't be surprised if…"

In the natural we are taught and conditioned to expect the worse so if something good happens, we are pleasantly surprised. The bad seems to be the norm, and the good an unexpected occurrence. But we shouldn't be surprised, because it's just the Kingdom principle in action. What you believe, you receive. What you gravitate towards, gravitates towards you. If you surround yourself with negativity, whether people, thoughts or results, negativity will surround and take over you.

If this is true, then the opposite must be true! It is not just a matter of having positive people and thoughts. Remember that as believers we have all of Heaven on our side and the Holy

Spirit on the inside! Our spirit is in conversation with Him as we read His Word, speak it out loud to increase our faith, and the Spirit imparts revelation to us from above.

God's Word is absolute truth! What it says, it will do. All we must do is take His Word into our minds (read it) and download it into our spirits (meditate on it). There the Holy Spirit begins to activate the power already inside to bring about miraculous change as daily we live out and speak the Word by faith.

This is a 100 percent spiritual guarantee; no 50/50 here! This is God we are dealing with, and His Word is always absolute truth! "He sent His Word and healed them" (Psalm 107:20). Therefore, I am healed! And I'm all in!

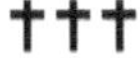

Reach Out
and Touch Him

March 13, 2015 (Friday)

Matthew 14:35-36 — *And when the men of that place recognized Him, they sent out into all that surrounding region, brought to Him all who were sick, and begged Him that they might only touch the hem of His garment. And as many as touched it were made perfectly well.*

✝✝✝

I believed in the Tooth Fairy. It was exciting to put my little tooth under the pillow and find a quarter in the morning. Then there was Santa Claus. Of course he was real and could make enough toys for all the children in the world. And without a doubt, he, Rudolph and the rest of the reindeer would make that incredible trip around the world to every house and climb down every chimney to leave presents and fill stockings. How could that not be true? He's Santa, for goodness sake!

Childlike faith believes the "impossible" to be possible, overriding laws of nature by the power and authority of the Truth given by the highest court of all existence to the Judge of all. And He, in turn, has given us access to that same power and authority. We can override laws of sickness and death by speaking and believing the Word of Truth. Nothing to figure out; and we don't have to have the answers or the means to make it happen. We just have to believe and know in our hearts and minds that it will happen!

The Tooth Fairy and Santa Claus are fairy tales. God is real, and He really wants me well and whole! So, Holy Spirit, come and take away all my doubts and fears and leave me with more faith, more perseverance, more power and Your wisdom. Please order my steps and establish me. Please reveal Yourself to me and show me, in Your timing, my destiny, my story that was written before the foundations of the world were made.

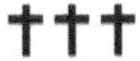

9

Binding and Loosing

March 14, 2015 (Saturday)

MATTHEW 18:18 — *Assuredly, I say to you, whatever you bind on earth will be bound in heaven, and whatever you loose on earth will be loosed in heaven.*

✝✝✝

"My people perish because of lack of knowledge" (Hosea 4:6). I was always taught to bind the negative or evil and loose the good or positive. But according to Matthew 18:18 (see Deuteronomy 6:4-9), it is just the opposite. Bind to the good—God's Word. Loose from the bad—all that is hindering me from a life of wholeness and abundance in Jesus Christ (see John 11, where Lazarus is loosed from graveclothes). Entwine my spirit with God's Spirit; interlock with Him until I have the mind and ways of Christ and power to do even greater works (John 14:12; Mark 16:17).

I just prayed for the pain under my rib cage that has been ongoing for over a week now by binding to God's Word and loosing it out of my body. The pain is gone in Jesus' name! This revelation is why the enemy didn't want me to do today's lesson.

Today I also literally stepped out on faith. My foot was hurting me so bad that I couldn't put any pressure on it. But I prayed and walked on it by faith, the pain left, and I was able to tutor, wash clothes, help Nana, etc.

Thank You; thank You, Lord!

I rest in Your Word, Lord. From this day forth, I will rest in Your Word. I am healed. I am healthy. I am whole!

Hear God. Agree with God. Speak that which you have heard.

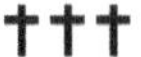

10

A Merry Heart

March 15, 2015 (Sunday)

Proverbs 17:22 — *A merry heart does good, like medicine, / But a broken spirit dries the bones.*

✝✝✝

We are tri-symbiotic beings: spirit, soul and body. If the three do not find a balance, the individual will cease to exist on the earth. The spirit is our life source from God; the soul is our mind, will and emotions; and the body holds both within—treasures in earthen vessels (2 Corinthians 4:7).

The body is a sensory entity; the spirit, a spiritual entity; and the two fight to rule the soul in this life and for eternity. Each wants to dominate. And let's not forget the spirit of Satan that uses our bodies to hijack our spirit and overtake our soul. Therefore, our spirit must agree with the Spirit of God to access His wisdom and power to counteract the attacks of the devil and to control the urges of our flesh.

The parts that make up our being are so intertwined that the physical affects the spiritual and the spiritual affects the physical. A depressive thought can make you feel tired or weak. A physical ailment can depress you and send your mind spiraling down.

God knew this and planned on our behalf. Proverbs 17:22 states, "A merry heart doeth good like a medicine." We take medicine to change the condition of our bodies. God prescribes a merry heart. Laughter produces chemicals in the body "that naturally boost the immune system," which God created "to fight every disease known to man" (Bowers, 108). The physical act of laughing affects us spiritually and psychologically, offering us a philosophical conversation on healing and restoration.

And according to the Word of God, "a broken spirit drieth the bones." The spirit depressed and in disarray affects the physical body and may destroy its potential or kill it. Therefore, let us always strive to agree with the Spirit of God. We do this through His Word. Hear It! Say It! Do It!

Choose life. Live, laugh, and enjoy. Laugh and be healed!

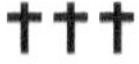

11

Don't Try to Figure It Out

March 16, 2015 (Monday)

PROVERBS 3:7-8 — *Do not be wise in your own eyes; / Fear the* LORD *and depart from evil. / It will be health to your flesh, / And strength to your bones.*

✝✝✝

I need to, and I will, fear the Lord. I will honor and respect Him, worship and adore Him. I will venerate my God, for He is worthy! I will reverence and glorify my God because of His supreme worth. Honor and high praise belong to Him, and Him alone. I will magnify Him and His holy name, extol and hold Him in greater esteem and respect. I will intensify my praise and adoration towards my God. I choose to love Him with all my body, heart, soul and spirit. I acknowledge His omnipotence.

This sensory world, with its evil intentions, will desensitize us to the reality of God and His power. We have eaten so much fruit from the Tree of Knowledge of Good and Evil that we are no longer able to even swallow a mustard seed of faith. We are trapped by the gravity of sickness and depression to the point where we can't mount up on wings like eagles, run and not get weary, walk and not faint (Isaiah 40:31).

Healing is the children's bread (Mark 7:24-30), and I am His child! I will eat of His Word, not from the Tree of the Knowledge of Good and Evil. I will fear Him! I will acknowledge Who

He is and seek His face! He is my Saviour; He is my Lord! If I do these things, it will be health to my navel and marrow to my bones!

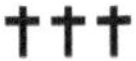

Refuse to Be Condemned

March 17, 2015 (Tuesday)

ROMANS 8:1 — *There is therefore now no condemnation to those who are in Christ Jesus, who do not walk according to the flesh, but according to the Spirit.*

†††

The past is the past. I have asked for forgiveness. Therefore, I am forgiven. "If we confess our sins, He is faithful and just to forgive us our sins and to cleanse us from all unrighteousness" (1 John 1:9). The Word *says* so; so it *is* so!

It is my desire to run towards God's Spirit and align myself with and bind myself to His Word so that when the Spirit opens the door to my healing manifestation, I will be ready to walk into that new dimension of Divine Health and Wholeness, which was purchased for me on Calvary by my Saviour and Lord, Jesus Christ. Until that happens, I will do my best with the help of the Lord to:

1. Seek God's face every day and commune with Him.

2. Learn and practice the biblical principles that will bring about my healing manifestation.

3. Develop my faith so that it is operational in the dimension where my covenant of health and wholeness resides.

4. Take care of my physical body through rest, exercise and good eating habits.

And if I fall short on any given day, I will not condemn myself, because "there is therefore now no condemnation."

I run towards You, Lord.

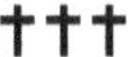

13

He Is Willing to Heal You

March 18, 2015 (Wednesday)

MATTHEW 8:2-3 — *And behold, a leper came and worshiped Him, saying, "Lord, if You are willing, You can make me clean." Then Jesus put out His hand and touched him, saying, "I am willing; be cleansed." Immediately his leprosy was cleansed.*

✝✝✝

God is not a genie in a bottle waiting to grant our requests or a magician with a magic wand. He wants us to live fulfilled, abundant lives and have the desires of our hearts; but buying our love is not how we receive from Him. He already paid the price for our lives at Calvary. He gave His best and His all because He loved us so much, and He offers Himself to us freely. He only asks for relationship in return. As He has committed to us, He only asks commitment to Him. He gives us His love and devotion, and He asks for the same.

Because of what God has done, we acknowledge Him for Who He is. We worship and fear Him because He is worthy— our Creator, Saviour, Protector, Loyal Friend, Brother, Lord and Guide—our Everything. And when we worship and delight ourselves in Him, He returns to us His love, peace, joy, kindness, and goodness through His Spirit and gladly meets all our needs and sometimes our wants. It is His desire for us to be happy. He just asks that we build a relationship with Him through worship.

Tonight started the Women's Department three-day revival. Evangelist Sybil Finney talked about how we are a blessed people of God, delighting in and meditating on His Word, chosen and predestined, God protecting and blessing us. Then we blessed the Lord at the altar, worshiping Him for Who He is and has been in our lives; not asking for anything, but blessing Him because He continuously blesses us.

What a confirmation of day thirteen. Worshiping puts us in position for God's Spirit to bless our spirit, situations, needs and wants. When we enter relationship with our God, no good thing is withheld from us. He loves us, and it is His desire to bless us. So, in turn, I will bless the Lord with all my heart, soul and mind and love Him just the same.

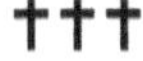

14

Remember the Sabbath

March 20, 2015 (Friday)

EXODUS 20:8-11 — *Remember the Sabbath day, to keep it holy. Six days you shall labor and do all your work, but the seventh day is the Sabbath of the LORD your God. In it you shall do no work: you, nor your son, nor your daughter, nor your male servant, nor your female servant, nor your cattle, nor your stranger who is within your gates. For in six days the LORD made the heavens and the earth, the sea, and all that is in them, and rested the seventh day. Therefore the LORD blessed the Sabbath day and hallowed it.*

✝✝✝

Have you ever been around someone that just won't be quiet? You're trying to relax and take in the moment, and they won't stop talking. Perhaps God feels that way. I've always thought that communing with Him consisted of talking to Him, telling Him how I feel about Him, asking Him to lead and guide me, asking for forgiveness, needs and wants, and then waiting for Him to respond to everything, or at least one thing.

Never did I think that a long, relaxing drive or stopping to take pictures along the way was just as much a time of communion as verbal dialogue. I used to think that I had failed at my time with Him and needed to talk more and focus my every thought towards Him. But now I am free from my misappropriated guilt. The exhale that takes place when I see His beauty before me, or when I experience the sunset that is new each and every day, to see the moonlight shine across the snow or a quiet midnight drive on "Canopy Road"—that is He and I communing in my soul.

The freedom and quiet that speak to my spirit from His, renewing me, quieting me—this *is* my Sabbath rest with Him; sacred moments shared with my Creator offering me His peace and healing if I will only be quiet and listen to His silence.

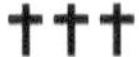

15

Your Life Is in Your Mouth

March 21, 2015 (Saturday)

PROVERBS 18:21 — *Death and life are in the power of the tongue, / And those who love it will eat its fruit.*

PROVERBS 12:18 — *There is one who speaks like the piercings of a sword, / But the tongue of the wise promotes health.*

✝✝✝

I have found it difficult to write my thoughts for day fifteen, "Your Life Is in Your Mouth." I believe that to be true, and it is so much more. The Bible says, "For as he thinketh in his heart, so is he" (Proverbs 23:7). And Luke 6:45 says, "Out of the abundance of the heart his mouth speaks." The word we speak starts as a thought, a seed, and gets rooted and grows in our hearts. How does it grow? By what we feed it. Do we feed it God's Word or with thoughts from our own mind? Do we water it daily with doubt or faith? Do we let the light of God's truth shine on it or let the clouds of man's limitation hover, blocking the one and only true Son?

When those words produce fruit, they become the fruit of our lips, which "is the natural outgrowth of the heart" (http:// www.desiringgod.org/messages/the-sacrifice-of-praise – "The Cultivation of Hearts Standing in Awe of God"). We speak them into the atmosphere; they break through into the spiritual realm, where they are echoed back to us; and we receive either blessings or cursings, life or death.

Words are powerful. It is not just what we say, but how we say it, that determines our level of faith, confidence, and conviction:

> "*You* can make it?" It's a joke.
> "You *can* make it." It's a possibility.
> "*You Can Make It!*" It's a belief.

"I can do all things through Christ who strengthens me" (Philippians 4:13) is a *decree*, an official order given by a person of authority usually having the force of law. In this case, the authority is through Jesus Christ. What law? God's law, "calling things that aren't as though they are" (Romans 4:17).

I must believe what I allow to be planted in my heart, feed and nurture it daily with God's Word, water it with faith, let the light of His Spirit shine on it, and watch it take root and grow in my spirit until it produces into the fruit of my lips (Hebrews 13:15; Proverbs 12:14), producing praise to God, healing and wholeness.

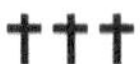

16

Settle All Doubts

March 23, 2015 (Monday)

Numbers 23:19 — *God is not a man, that He should lie, / Nor a son of man, that He should repent. / Has He said, and will He not do? / Or has He spoken, and will He not make it good?*

✝✝✝

Faith: "The *substance* of things *hoped* for, the evidence of things not seen" (Hebrews 11:1).

Substance: Essence; the ultimate reality that *underlies* all outward manifestations and change.

Underlies: Forms the basis or foundation of an idea, process, etc.

Hope: To want something to happen or be true and think that it is possible; to cherish a desire with anticipation, expectation or *obtainment*; to expect with confidence or trust.

Obtainment: To gain or attain, usually by planned action or effort; to realize, capture; to cause to become real; to achieve your desire.

Cherish: To keep and cultivate a desire with care and affection; to entertain or harbor in the mind deeply, resolutely, with determination.

All Outward Manifestations: Thymus gland, lungs, liver, gallbladder, autoimmune disease, lymphatic system, vocal cords, eyes, all other organs and systems.

"Faith is the substance of things hoped for, the evidence of things not seen" (Hebrews 11:1). "Faith cometh by hearing and hearing by the Word of God" (Romans 10:17). Faith in God's Word, which is The Truth, is the ultimate reality that we stand on. It is the foundation on which all that we desire rests and is realized. We keep and cultivate that desire with care and affection. We harbor it in our minds deeply, with great determination, with a do-or-die mentality, with anticipation and expectation, with confidence and trust in God.

By reading and meditating on God's Word, we internalize it until it takes root and blossoms into the fruit of our lips and we eat thereof and sing. We live in its truth until our spirit-man and the Spirit of Truth align to produce the gateway to the dimension of Divine Health and Wholeness and we take the key of faith that unlocks the door where we shall find the reality of it all.

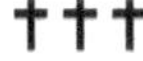

17

The Love Factor

March 24, 2015 (Tuesday)

John 17:23 — *...That the world may know that You have sent Me, and have loved them as You have loved Me.*

†††

Thank You, God, for loving me as You do Your Son! I never knew that or didn't have the spiritual discernment to comprehend it. But my spirit-man heard it and embraced it. If you had asked me if I thought God loved me, I would have said, "Yes, of course He does!" But if you had asked me if He loved me as much as He loves Jesus, I would have said, "Of course not! Let's not get ridiculous!"

But the unbelievable truth is He does! Jesus said it in John 17:23 as He was talking to His Father. It was important to Him that we comprehend it: "That the world may know that Thou hast sent Me and hast loved them as Thou hast loved Me." But even more than this, according to John 5:19 and 12:49, these words are from the very mouth and will of God!

John 5:19 – "Very truly I tell you, the Son can do nothing by himself; he can do only what he sees his Father doing, because whatever the Father does the Son also does" (NIV).

John 12:49 – "For I did not speak on my own, but the Father who sent me commanded me to say all that I have spoken" (NIV).

God is the very essence of love; and He loved us so much that He came to us in the Person of His Son, Jesus Christ. He sent all His love, the best of Himself:

- To heal us, spirit, mind and body, and ransom our souls to have abundant and eternal life;
- To be heirs and joint-heirs with Christ forever;
- To share in the promise to Abraham's descendants, adopted into the family of God, brothers and sisters of Christ, friends;
- To give us His power—the same Spirit that raised Jesus from the dead—to quicken, lead and guide us, to fight the good fight of faith, to break down the strongholds of the enemy, and to be a light to lead those that are lost to the path of life.

God has given us all rights and privileges, His love and His power, as though we were His own Son! What more can He do? It is up to us to believe and receive all that the Divine has in store for us. I start with His love!

Thank You, God, for loving me as You do Your Son!

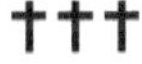

18

Be Thankful

March 26, 2015 (Thursday)

1 THESSALONIANS 5:18 — *In everything give thanks; for this is the will of God in Christ Jesus for you.*

✝✝✝

It is easy to succumb to the leading of the flesh governed by the five senses: seeing, hearing, smelling, tasting, and touching. Our spirit is encased within the body, which unfortunately becomes the first defense to the sensitivity of the spirit. The Spirit asks us to see with our spiritual eyes of faith when nothing is there. Our natural eyes consider that to be blindness. When our bodies are racked with pain, and we feel depressed and rejected by God, the Spirit says in all things give thanks and call things that are not as though they are (Romans 4:17).

Our natural minds can't comprehend these things. God's ways and thoughts are "as far as the east is from the west" (cf. Isaiah 55:8-9; Psalm 103:8-12). Life is a continuous journey of growth and maturity. We only reach our destiny through trials and difficulties that build our character and build up our spirit-man, which enables us to grow in the knowledge of God and the fear of the Lord, which is the beginning of wisdom (Psalm 111:10).

And God said that He would multiply my days and add years to my life if I would acknowledge Him (cf. Proverbs 9:10-11). So I thank God for all things. It opens the gates to Him, where

He blesses and heals me. And I grow and learn and become everything that God created me to be.

So I thank Him for all the mountains. They take me to a higher place, a holy place. There I enter His gates (Psalm 100:4), and I am healed.

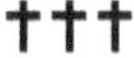

19
Get Your Prayer Strategy Right

March 27, 2015 (Friday)

2 PETER 1:3-4 — *As His divine power has given to us all things that pertain to life and godliness, through the knowledge of Him who called us by glory and virtue, by which have been given to us exceedingly great and precious promises, that through these you may be partakers of the divine nature.*

✝✝✝

We are spirit. Therefore our words are spirit, and they come from the depths of our souls. They are never just idle words; they come with a purpose and the power to execute their intent.

There is only evil and good in the world; so our words will be for evil or for good. What we speak we will have. Our words carry through sound waves, creating echoes that break through our atmosphere into the spiritual realm, creating gateways to the throne of God or passageways into the darkness of evil. Our words carry weight or light through their meaning.

Words make deep roots where planted. The sower waits with great anticipation to see what harvest will come. So my words are my harvest. When I speak the Word of the Lord over my life through prayer in every situation, it produces His healing throughout my being. If my words give life to my pains and problems, they will overtake me like weeds, and I am lost.

The choice is mine. I am the prophet over my life. I acknowledge my circumstance but place full confidence in the power of God as I speak His Word into my situation. The strategy is to always speak His words of healing, life and power. His words, filled with faith and hope, must always enter the atmosphere. Like a machine gun, His words must riddle through the air, destroying the enemy of doubt, sickness, disease, and pain as we scream our battle cry:

"By the power vested in me, by the Blood of Jesus Christ, I say to you, (*name the condition*), it is written, (*name the healing*), in Jesus' name. AMEN!"

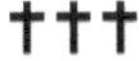

20
Little by Little

March 30, 2015 (Monday)

Exodus 23:30 — *By little and little I will drive them out from before you, until you have increased, and you inherit the land.*

✝✝✝

Today I woke up with symptoms of being overtired and improper airflow into my lungs. I have had these symptoms before; and in the past I have either scheduled an impromptu visit to the hospital to get my blood checked or have felt a panic attack begin. In one episode this past year, I drove myself to the emergency room because I panicked and felt like I was about to pass out.

But today I used the new method that I have been taught by taking God's medicine, His Word, to fight everything that rises against me and appropriate my healing manifestation. I calmly spoke the Word of God out loud; and by faith through my spirit-man, we aligned with the Spirit—the same Spirit that raised Jesus from the dead that lives inside of me—and He quickened my body (Romans 8:11).

I know that I must get more rest and implement exercise into my life; but today I took a giant step in the right direction—a step waiting to happen since 2002. My breathing is better than it was when I woke up. I don't feel wiped out. I don't need to go to the hospital. The power of God's Word has healed my symptoms; and I move forward in His healing virtue, step by step, little by little, until I walk into the fullness of my healing manifestation.

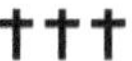

21

Can I Fix It?

March 30, 2015 (Monday)

GALATIANS 6:7 — *Do not be deceived, God is not mocked; for whatsoever a man sows, that he will also reap.*

✝✝✝

I believe it was a coach from the Stanford's Division 1 women's basketball team who told her players, "If you want things you never had before, you have to do things you've never done before." Conversely, if you do things the same way, expect to get the same results. It's not rocket science. Whenever you add 1+1, no matter what, you will always get 2.

My issue with getting the proper amount of rest started in high school. My schedule was extremely busy with commuting, after-school sports, homework, and much stress. I was up until the early morning hours every night, neglecting my body. This carried over into college and into adulthood, abusing my body through various means. And since I was diagnosed in 2002, along with all that I have endured for the past thirteen years, sleep has not come easy or often.

My efforts get high marks for good intentions, but I fail miserably at putting those good intentions into action. I do not want to block my own manifestation. I have come too far to be my worst enemy. I realize that repentance is not just saying "I'm sorry." It is the action required in response to saying "I'm sorry."

Please forgive me, Lord, for my inaction. I admit my inability to solve this issue in my life; and I ask You, Holy Spirit, to take control. I surrender all of this and all of me to You. Please help me to not be afraid to lie down in peace and sweet sleep:

Proverbs 3:24 – When you lie down, you will not be afraid; when you lie down, your sleep will be sweet.

Psalm 4:8 – I will both lie down in peace and sleep; for You alone, O LORD, make me dwell in safety.

Thank You, Trinity, for hearing my prayer; for You are my Shepherd, and I shall not want. You make me lie down in green pastures, You lead me beside still waters, You restore my soul (Psalm 23:1-3).

✝✝✝

I also call Susan I been watching [Joy added this line while transcribing the entries from her journal to computer. There is no other mention to clarify this.]

22

No Disease Is Too Hard for Jesus

March 31, 2015 (Tuesday)

MATTHEW 4:23 — *And Jesus went about all Galilee, teaching in their synagogues, preaching the gospel of the kingdom, and healing all kinds of sickness and all kinds of disease among the people.*

†††

There was always that class in school that was harder than the rest. It demanded more time, more study, total focus and full attention to detail. It was the course you needed to pass. No shortcuts or alternatives. No other way to get to the next level. It was not an elective. Your future depended on it. Long hours preparing for each pop quiz and test. Never missing a lecture, keywords were committed to memory so that during the final exam, you could answer all questions and silence any doubts that the requirements to pass the course were indeed fulfilled. And after all the demands, the all-nighters, in-depth conversations and contemplations, you were tested, you were tried. So...

1. Read the Manual or Manuscript
2. Listen carefully to the Instructor
3. Follow the directions
4. Study hard, study long. You can't go wrong.

For some, it will come easy; for others, it will take time. Just stay the course; don't give up. You will find your way and graduate at the top of your class. Nothing is too hard for God. You're rollin' with Him!

"Take My yoke upon you, and learn of Me;…for My yoke is easy and My burden is light" (Matthew 11:29-30). Graduation day is coming!

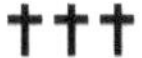

23
God Watches Over His Word

April 1, 2015 (Wednesday)

ISAIAH 55:11 — *So shall My word be that goes forth from My mouth; / It shall not return to Me void, / But it shall accomplish what I please, / And it shall prosper in the thing for which I sent it.*

JEREMIAH 1:12 — *Then the LORD said to me, "You have seen well, for I am ready to perform My word."*

✝✝✝

"Work with me." At times when I have been low energy and not feeling 100 percent, my mother has spoken these words as she stepped in to help me, to lighten my load, because physically I couldn't handle things. It meant she was going to put forth most of the effort, but I still had to do my part regardless how small it might be. It was a team effort; and even if I could only give 10 percent, neither of us was going to do the task alone.

I hear God saying the same thing, "Work with Me." He is going to make sure that my healing takes place. He is watching over His Word to perform it, to make sure that it does what He says. There is no question of the outcome; that was settled over 2,000 years ago. So that just leaves me then. As Ms. Freeda says, you have to give Him something to work with. I am beginning to understand that more as the forty days continue.

For God to perform His Word, there has to be a Word there. Where? In the air! We work between a spiritual and a physical world. The plans and laws have already been established. The plan is for us to read and speak God's Word back to Him. The law is that faith and belief must be present for us to receive our manifestation from God. When those things are in place, the plan ends with our receiving healing and wholeness because the law says that God's Word goes forth, never to return to Him void. It will accomplish what He pleases and will prosper in the thing for which He sent it.

Psalm 107:20 – He sent His Word and healed them.

3 John 1:2 – Beloved, I pray that you may prosper in all things, and be in health, as your soul prospers.

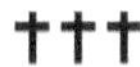

24

Possess What Belongs to You

April 3, 2015 (Friday)

Joshua 1:3 — *Every place that the sole of your foot will tread upon I have given you.*

✝✝✝

[STILL A WORK IN PROGRESS]
This is the service that I want to have after my healing is fully manifested. Working through this thoughtfully.

CELEBRATION OF LIFE!
Service of Healing and Thanksgiving
Service of Thanksgiving and Wholeness

Songs: "Faith" by Andre Crouch
"Sho'Nuff" by Hezekiah Walker

Call to Worship: Rev. Marilyn Lambe

"This is the day that the Lord has made; we will rejoice and be glad in it!" (Psalm 118:24)

"I will say of the Lord, 'He is my refuge and my fortress, my God, in whom I trust.'" (Psalm 91:2)

"O magnify the Lord with me; let us exalt His name together!" (Psalm 34:3)

✝✝✝

Joy's mother, Reverend Marilyn Lambe, remembers Joy's anticipation for a celebration of her healing:

> *"Mom, I want you to be the worship leader. We will invite the doctors, nurses and all who were involved in my healing. Uncle Robert will preach and tell them about the healing power of God."*

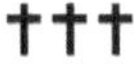

25

Ask What Ye Will

April 4, 2015 (Saturday)

JOHN 15:7 — *If you abide in Me, and My words abide in you, you will ask what you desire, and it shall be done for you.*

✝✝✝

3+4 will always equal 7. I don't care what you do; forever and always 3+4 will equal 7. That is the order of things. Math is an exact science; and though dividing numbers can result in repeating decimals that never end, when we add two whole numbers, we get a sum that is totally dependent upon the addends. Whatever the two addends, they determine the sum; and the sum can't be any more or less than the two addends. The three are forever bound together.

Just as it is with numbers, how much more it is with the Word of God. What it says, it means. What it says to do, we must do to get the results it promises. There are no repeating decimals, no shortcuts or options to choose from. If you fulfill the demands or requirements, you will achieve the goal. If you don't, you won't. As my grandfather used to say, "It may be tight, but it's right!" Easy to comprehend, yet much discipline to implement and diligence to continue are required until the goal is achieved and the victory is won.

John 15:7 – If you abide in Me [the first addend +], and My Words abide in you [the second addend=], you *shall* ask what you will, and it *shall* be done unto you.

Revelation: The sum is in the future tense! It is a done deal! You are going to ask what you will, and you will have it!

Lord, help me to add up enough of Your Presence and Your Words so that the sum is Healing and Wholeness!

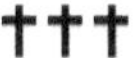

26

Stop Signing for the Package

April 5, 2015 (Easter Sunday)

HEBREWS 4:14-15 — *Seeing then that we have a great High Priest who has passed through the heavens, Jesus the Son of God, let us hold fast our confession. For we do not have a High Priest who cannot sympathize with our weaknesses.*

✝✝✝

My senses have been testifying, but I refuse to say "Amen." There is a fight going on between my physical body and my spirit-man. My body is out of alignment. Holy Spirit, align my spirit with Yours so that my body will be drawn into the open portal of Divine Healing and Wholeness. My body is trying to reject the "Medicine" that I am daily pouring in as though it has the right to "Return to Sender." But my spirit-man is in control as led by the Holy Spirit; and we have decided that no matter what, God's Word is more powerful than any pain or symptoms that my body tries to submit as the true reality in my life.

All pain, symptoms and negative thoughts are going to be "Returned to Sender." My new reality is that we are going to do exactly what the Word says. "If you abide in Me, and My Words abide in you, you shall ask what you will and it shall be given unto you" (John 15:7). There is only *one* reality.

1. I will not die, but live and proclaim the works of the Lord. (Psalm 118:17)

2. Life and death are in the tongue. (Proverbs 18:21)

3. I choose life!

4. No weapon formed against me shall prosper. (Isaiah 54:17)

5. Greater is He that is within me than he that is in the world. (1 John 4:4)

6. It is the same Spirit that raised Jesus from the dead that lives inside of me to quicken my mortal body. (Romans 8:11)

7. Bless the Lord, O my soul; and all that is within me, bless His holy name. Bless the Lord, O my soul, and forget not all His benefits, Who:

    i. Heals my diseases
    ii. Redeems my soul from destruction
    iii. Forgives my sins
    iv. Crowns me with loving-kindness and
    v. Tender mercies
    vi. Satisfies my mouth with good things
    vii. So that my youth is renewed like the eagle's (Psalm 103:1-5)

8. Beloved, I pray that you prosper in all things and be in health, as your soul prospers. (3 John 1:2)

9. So shall My Word be that goes forth out of My mouth. It shall not return to me void, but shall accomplish what I please and prosper in why I sent it. (Isaiah 55:11)

10. He sent His Word and healed them. (Psalm 107:20)

11. By Whose stripes I was healed!!! (1 Peter 2:24)

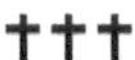

27
Guard Your Heart
April 7, 2015 (Tuesday)

PROVERBS 4:23 — *Keep your heart with all diligence, / For out of it spring the issues of life.*

✝✝✝

The dichotomous nature of being spirit and flesh can only be controlled and balanced by a disciplined life lived through the Spirit of God. However, it is through the five senses that we receive and deposit into our spirit. Therefore, what comes out of our spirit is exactly what we have allowed in. It's a choice; it's free will. God's Spirit longs to pour into us; and the process is interactive. "Faith without works is dead" (James 2:20). The way God pours into us is that we listen to His living, tangible Word, read and speak His Word, and then apply it to our lives by doing what it says to do. When we do that, what comes out will be "rivers of living water," which equals the Spirit in all its manifest power through the laying on of hands (healing), prophesy and answered prayer.

John 7:38 – He that believeth on me, as the scripture hath said, out of his belly shall flow rivers of living water.

John 4:14 – But whosoever drinketh of the water that I shall give him shall never thirst; but the water that I shall give him shall be in him a well of water springing up into everlasting life.

If we don't allow God's Spirit in, evil in its many forms and variants comes in; and what comes out is diabolical in nature.

That is why we must guard our heart with all diligence—minute to minute, moment to moment. It is crucial to our survival and well-being.

We are a living paradox: dichotomous and symbiotic at the same time. And we can live in perfect harmony if we choose. I choose life through the Spirit of God.

Holy Spirit, help me to censor everything that desires to enter into my being and only allow what is pleasing and acceptable in Your sight, that will benefit me spiritually and physically, that I may be enabled, empowered and equipped to fulfill the purposed destiny that You created just for me—through, with and in Your power and wisdom. Amen.

✝✝✝

Note: This is the last journal entry Joy transcribed from her notebook to computer. When she transcribed the first twenty-seven entries, she divided them into paragraphs, which were not in her handwritten originals. The last thirteen journal entries, which were transcribed after her transitioning, have no paragraph breaks.

28

Send the Invitation

April 9, 2015 (Thursday)

Jeremiah 33:3 — *Call to Me, and I will answer you, and show you great and mighty things, which you do not know.*

†††

In the Old Testament, when one entered the temple, there were three levels of entry: the Outer Court, the Inner Court and the Holy of Holies, where only the high priest was allowed to enter. That was the most sacred place, where the Spirit of God resided. Now, because of Jesus and His great sacrifice, we are no longer limited to the "outer court." We can enter into the Holy of Holies through our own hearts because the same Spirit that raised Jesus from the dead lives in us (Romans 8:9-11).… The Holy Spirit is there waiting for me to be free of all the busyness of the world so that I am at full liberty to commune with Him. I must give Him my full attention and reverence. He is God; how and why would I not? I don't know Him like I should. I don't trust Him like I should. I don't love Him like I should. It's all about relationship! I need relationship with my God, Creator, Saviour, Friend.… He said to call Him and He would answer and show me, not just tell me, great and mighty things that I know not of. What an invitation! How can I not accept? He is calling me. I am answering. It really is an open invitation. I am entering the first level, and He is calling me to rest. He is preparing me for what I know not of. It will require all my energy, strength, my faculties, my spirit aligned to His.... So now I rest....

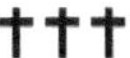

29

Did God Make Me Sick?

April 11, 2015 (Saturday)

Deuteronomy 28:61 — *Also every sickness and every plague, which is not written in this Book of the Law, will the Lord bring upon you until you are destroyed.*

✝✝✝

Did God make me sick? If you had asked me that question in the past, I would have said yes. Why yes? Because He was trying to get my attention or trying to teach me something. It is interesting that correctly translating Deuteronomy 28:61 by using a permissive verb instead of a causative one can still produce a sickness or disease in one's body; but the reasoning behind it makes all the difference. God is not intentionally sending disease and affliction. He destroyed that over 2,000 years ago when Jesus was whipped and endured thirty-nine strikes. Sometimes He allows the enemy to afflict us, as in Job's case; and sometimes we ourselves open that door. In my case, I believe I opened that door. I ran my body amuck. I had lost total control, and I was headed down a dark path of no return. Though God allowed my affliction, I give all honor and praise to Him because in His Word it says that what the devil means for harm God can turn around for my good (Genesis 50:20; Romans 8:28). What the enemy thought would do me in stopped me in my tracks and forced me off the dark path I was blindly on. It forced me into the path of light. Though still blinded, I am not alone and am allowing myself to be led by the Holy Spirit. I am on the path of life now with a hope and a future. It is God, in His infinite wisdom, that I am learning to trust. Allowing my affliction has made my destiny sure. Allowing this valley assures one day for me a mountaintop. Blessed be the name of the Lord! Thank you, Lord!

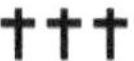

Divine Healing Vs. Divine Health

April 12, 2015 (Sunday)

REVELATIONS 12:11 — *And they overcame him by the blood of the Lamb and by the word of their testimony.*

✝✝✝

Living in the "glow" of His Glory, where sickness and disease cannot exist; that's where I want to be—in Divine Health. It was early in summer, and I was all alone kneeling in a hump on the kitchen floor. I had reached an end of eight years of pain marked by self-induced smiles. Now the mask had cracked open, and all the pain of those eight years began to pour out in tears on that kitchen floor. "Help me; please help me," I cried. It was my spirit-man crying out from the depths of my soul, held hostage by a body, held hostage by the destroyer of my soul. I did not know where to go, but I did know who to call. Not knowing if He would answer me, I called from the bottom of my soul. And then in an instant, without warning or a feeling coming on, I was engulfed in this presence, a spiritual realm of peace and healing. My eyes no longer teared—like the Israelites crossing the Red Sea on dry land. My pain no longer existed, and I was suspended in the flow of His Glory, floating on His healing wings, lovingly held in His arms. It was peace that passes all understanding (Philippians 4:7); it was God shall wipe all tears from their eyes (Revelation 21:4). It was my God offering healing to me—healing for my whole being, for everything in that moment was healed. In that moment, I was set free. It was the "glow" of His Glory. The portal had been opened, and I was invited in. Now I long for that moment again, but this time to stay and live in the "glow" of His Glory, in His Divine Wholeness and Health.

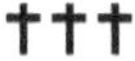

Confess Your Faults

April 14, 2015 (Tuesday)

JAMES 5:16 — *Confess your trespasses to one another, and pray for one another, that you may be healed. The effective, fervent prayer of a righteous man avails much.*

✝✝✝

When I scroll through the contacts in my phone, it is amazing to me just how many people there are. Six aggressive scrolls and the names keep rolling by, like the bonus wheel on "The Price Is Right." Names and businesses all in alphabetical order like I'm some big-time CEO. But the truth of the matter is, when I really think about who I would or could call in the wee hours of the morning when I really need to vent or reach out for help, outside of family, I find myself scrolling those same six times without stopping. Those contacts are the outer circle of my existence. Many have come and gone, and the ones that are still around are on the outskirts. I don't have an inner circle. I have no one to call, and no one calls me. No one to really confess to or pray with. My world is very, very quiet these days. And that probably isn't a bad thing. I am working on my relationship with God, and that demands all of my time. My need for others in the past has not served me well. My complete focus must be the Journey to My Destiny, a journey that will lead me to the realm of Divine Wholeness as guided by the Holy Spirit. Therefore, my spirit must always be in tune to hear and always aligned and ready to move when the Spirit moves. This is a journey meticulous in nature, requiring much patience and perseverance; no shortcuts or steps bypassed. It is a journey that requires careful interaction with others so as not to get sidetracked borrowing hours from the future with futile gain. So I look only to the Holy Spirit to confess my faults these days, as I wait patiently for my inner circle that only the Trinity has preordained. I look forward to that day. No more scrolling to see a random name appear; for there is no randomness with God, no happenstance. Before I call, they will have already answered (Isaiah 65:24); and what I need will have already been given. It's already done; the plan is complete. I just must keep walking towards my destiny until I arrive at the open door and walk into the realm of Divine Wholeness, where my life abundant begins.

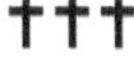

32

You Are Not Judge or Jury

April 18, 2015 (Saturday)

MATTHEW 6:14-15 — *For if you forgive men their trespasses, your heavenly Father will also forgive you. But if you do not forgive men their trespasses, neither will your Father forgive your trespasses.*

Colossians 3:13 — Bearing with one another, and forgiving one another, if anyone has a complaint against another; even as Christ forgave you, so you also must do.

✝✝✝

We are all God's masterpieces, yet all still works in progress. Still running the race, still trying to reach the goal. Still making mistakes, still fighting the flesh. We are human, both body and soul. No wings or glorified body, we live in a realm where there is a constant battle for our souls. Not all of us have the Holy Spirit living on the inside, our Resident God to lead and guide us and steer us away from wrong. Even with the Holy Spirit, we sometimes choose our own way and find ourselves in a place where we need forgiveness. We all fall, and sometimes we hurt the very ones that we are supposed to love, which means I could hurt you and you could hurt me. Deliberate or unbeknownst hurt can be inflicted; and sometimes we don't get those two words we need to make everything all right, "I'm sorry." And sometimes those words will never come. If we hold on to the pain and let it seep into our minds and filter into our hearts and attach its evil devices in our souls, it has the potential to detonate and destroy us. It's like the Blob and feeds on all the negativity around and grows and grows until it's no longer just pain but also anger and hate. God is love, and He only operates out of love. And if God is truly in me, I too must only emulate love. So there is no choice, no option. I must forgive even if I never hear "I'm sorry." I must do unto others as I would have them do unto me (Matthew 7:12). For God to forgive me, I must forgive and show unconditional love. Please help me, Lord. I want nothing between me and Thee. Holy Spirit, please lead and guide me into Your right paths. Help me to see myself and realize that I too have needed forgiveness, and still do. Let me always be sensitive to others, knowing that we are all human, God's masterpieces, still works in progress, still running the race, still trying to reach the goal, still in need of forgiveness.

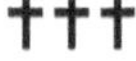

33

Healing Is in Your Mouth

April 20, 2015 (Monday)

Romans 10:8 — *"The word is near you, in your mouth and in your heart"* (that is, the word of faith which we preach).

†††

I heard the cock crow three times (cf. Mark 14:27ff). Yesterday I was working on a project that should have been easy and straightforward, but for some reason I ran into all kinds of problems. Nothing was working right; and in my frustration I said out loud, with no thought or reservation, "I can never catch a break!" My brother was on the phone, and he immediately said, "Watch what you say." I couldn't believe I had said it and immediately changed my words.… Today I had to parallel park on a street where cars were behind me. There was a car waiting to pull out in the space behind where I was going to park. I figured I would let him go and then I would have plenty of room to back in. Parallel parking has never been my favorite thing to do. But he blinked his lights, telling me to park; and I got real nervous and said something to the effect, "I can't do this! I'm the worst at this!" I immediately caught myself again and said something like, "I can do this! I'm good at this!" Then I turned the wheel and backed in—one of my best parking efforts.… During tutoring today, the bottom of my feet started aching; and when I stood up, the pain made it uncomfortable to walk. By the time I had dropped off my cousin, the aching was persistent. Out of my stress over the situation I said, "My feet are killing me!" Then I immediately said, "No, they aren't killing me!" And I began to proclaim the Word of God over my feet. And though the aching was still there and continues now, I told my body that it must line up with my spirit, which is aligned with the Spirit of God within me.… I have been going about this all wrong, trying to convince my body to line up and ascertain the things of the Spirit. It is my spirit that I should be focusing on—my spirit communing with God's Spirit, which resides inside of me; aligning myself to His Spirit so, like two magnets, the connection can never be repelled. Then my body will be drawn into alignment, like a total solar eclipse, ready for the manifestation of health and wholeness from the spiritual realm when the portal is opened. My words from the heart of my soul give light to my state of maturity in Christ and the level of my faith to believe and receive. Healing is the children's bread! Please, no more rooster's crow! I am ready. Try me again!

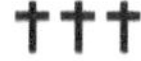

34

Be Led of the Spirit

April 27, 2015 (Monday)

GALATIANS 3:3 — *Are you so foolish? Having begun in the Spirit, are you now made perfect by the flesh?*

✝✝✝

Today has produced many confirmations in my life. On day thirty-three, I talked about going about this whole thing wrong—trying to get my natural man, which is my intellectual reasoning and physical body, to line up with the Spirit of God and what He and the living Word say. That is impossible! As far as the east is from the west so are His thoughts from ours (Isaiah 55:8-9; Psalm 103:8-12). It must be our spirit being led by the Spirit that produces results in our natural body. At our Women's Weekend service on Friday night, Evangelist Kennedy talked about how we move forward in God as a process. It is not like a microwave, but in many cases a slow, persistent process that teaches and perfects us in the ways and plan of God for our lives. The longer we spend time in the presence of God, the more we get to know Him, the more He is able to impart to us, the more power we gain to do that which He has called us to do. I want to be a leader in God's army that lives in and battles from the dimension of Divine Health and Wholeness. I want to live with a "Right Now Faith" mentality. Expecting the manifestations of the miraculous today, I surrender and yield, submitting my spirit to the Spirit of God. I align myself with only what He says and wants. I am willing to forgo my desires and follow where He leads. I know it is a process, a daily walk, a daily commitment. And I choose His way; I choose life—life in the Spirit, led by the Spirit, walking in the Spirit, moving forward into the spiritual realm of Divine Health and Wholeness, where I will live forever, showing the way for others to follow and to enter in the dimension where the Holy Spirit is and lives within.

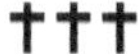

35

Hire the Guards

April 28, 2015 (Tuesday)

PHILIPPIANS 4:8 — *Finally, brethren, whatever things are true, whatever things are noble, whatever things are just, whatever things are pure, whatever things are lovely, whatever things are of good report, if there is any virtue and if there is anything praiseworthy—meditate on these things.*

✝✝✝

This verse is the litmus test of the power and integrity of my praise. The Pharisees accused the disciples of being unclean for not washing their hands before eating. Jesus quickly came to their defense and let the Pharisees know that what comes out is really what's dirty. It's not a natural thing but a spiritual thing. When we speak, the atmosphere is opened to the spiritual realm; and what we say dictates what happens there. Man looks at the outside appearance, but God looks at the heart (1 Samuel 16:7). And it is out of the heart that the mouth speaks (Matthew 12:34). What we think, our thoughts, are the seeds we plant; and when we meditate on them, we are giving life to those thoughts, whether good or bad; and they grow and produce fruit—"the fruit of our lips" (Hebrews 13:15). That's what we speak, what we say without even thinking, because that is what is in our hearts. Paul admonishes us in Philippians 4:8 to think on things that are TRUE, HONEST, JUST, PURE, LOVELY, OF GOOD REPORT. That is where true and real power lies and where we will find authentic praise. There is a release of God's power to produce positive change in our lives and circumstances. Praise and adoration directed to Him effects a change in the very atmosphere, in our environments, which will trigger noticeable change in every aspect of our being. And beware, this law works both ways. The test is whether what I say from my heart and my praise to God are in line with Philippians 4:8. If they are, I will see significant change and positive results physically, spiritually and emotionally in my life. If they're not, then it's time to "hire the guards," each with their own stack of litmus paper: TRUTH, HONESTY, JUSTICE, PURITY, LOVELINESS and GOOD REPORTS. Every thought, before it becomes spoken word, must pass through the paper; and if the color changes, I know that I must destroy that thought until my heart is as authentic as the praise I long to offer You.

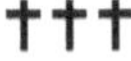

This page intentionally left blank.

36

Your Future Is Stored in Your Heart

April 30, 2015 (Thursday)

MATTHEW 12:35 — *A good man out of the good treasure of his heart brings forth good things, and an evil man out of the evil treasure brings forth evil things.*

✝✝✝

I have felt different in my spirit-man these days: lighter, freer, a buildup of faith. I have not conquered years of indiscipline; but I have been positively walking in the path of discipline, taking daily steps towards the health and wholeness portal door. I feel communion in my spirit with the Holy Spirit that lives within me. Every time I speak Jesus to my symptomatic body and believe, there is a release of healing virtue that must take place, because God honors His Word more than His very name. As gravity is a law of nature, so are the results of following God's Word a law of spiritual magnitude that will always be honored by God Himself. So I will continue in the way with a greater press and determination. I am in control, the prophet of my soul. How long will this take? How clear are my eyes of faith? Clear enough to see The Word? To speak The Word? To commune with The Word? To believe The Word? Yes! My resolve is clear and true; stay on the road; my destiny is near. Follow the Son, the light of the moon; just around the bend the portal door awaits me. I am ready to enter in.

✝✝✝

37

The Laying On of Hands

May 5, 2015 (Tuesday)

Luke 4:40 — *When the sun was setting, all those who had any that were sick with various diseases brought them to Him; and He laid His hands on every one of them and healed them.*

†††

I left Central Park with new revelation, a new understanding of the laying on of hands—the hand of God touching me. We are His point of contact. We are the temple where He lives, where He reigns. The same Spirit that raised Jesus from the dead lives in me to quicken my mortal body (Romans 8:11). In Him I live and move and have my being (Acts 17:28). He permeates and radiates from within me. Therefore when I touch someone in His name, that point of contact enables His power to pass through and prosper in the thing for which it was sent (Isaiah 55:11). My faith and belief, my spirit-man, must be aligned with His Spirit for the power to be released.… I was listening to healing scriptures this morning and fell into another realm of consciousness. I saw my Father reaching through the spiritual realm to me, His hand extending through the open portal door. I was nervous at first; it was so real, and I didn't know if it was true. But I made contact and felt a surge of healing virtue flow through one side of my body and then into the other. I felt healing and wellness. I was whole. I awoke into this realm of consciousness, for a moment wondering if my manifestation had come. Maybe it did; maybe it's here waiting for the natural man to embrace the manifestation inside. But all I know is that I felt the hand of God touch me, and I was whole. Therefore, I am whole. No more weapons shall prosper over me.

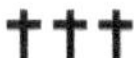

38

What Will You Wear?

May 10, 2015 (Sunday)

PHILIPPIANS 2:3 — *Let nothing be done through selfish ambition or conceit, but in lowliness of mind let each esteem others better than himself.*

✝✝✝

In the movie "The Ultimate Gift," a young man is put through a series of tests to receive the inheritance left for him by his grandfather. All the tests focused on helping others, being a friend, and being sensitive to the needs of others. Most of all the test was to give from his heart without reservation or an uncaring attitude. Having lived a spoiled, selfish life, these changes were hard to implement. He was used to using people and having his own way. But slowly he began to understand the blessings of service. He experienced what it means to touch someone's inner being in such a profound way, making such a great impact on their life, that the blessing rebounds to you and you are forever changed. This is exactly what happened to this young man. He gave all that he had to help others. He poured out of himself what was given to him with no thought of self-preservation or prideful aspirations. He went beyond what man would require. He entered the God realm, where denial, service and sacrifice are hallmarks of a life yielded to the Spirit. It is what God calls us to—a life of service to others through gifts, talents and passions so that they may fulfill what God has called them to. When we are obedient and do His will, there is nothing that He will withhold from us. He will pour down on us blessings that we cannot even fathom. We will be blessed exponentially. What was the ultimate gift? The billion-dollar inheritance he received after passing each test? No, it was what he learned and gained throughout the process: the joy and love he found that he never had before, and the inner peace and satisfaction that can only be found by doing what one was created to do: Love God and love your neighbor as yourself (Mark 12:30-31).

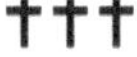

39

Thy Will Be Done

May 14, 2015 (Thursday)

MATTHEW 6:10 — *Your kingdom come. / Your will be done / On earth as it is in heaven.*

✝✝✝

Here we are, day thirty-nine. Full circle. Surrender. Thy will be done in earth and in me an earthen vessel, in the temple where You abide and reside—"treasure in earthen vessels" (2 Corinthians 4:7). I open my heart and my soul to You, Lord. Thy kingdom come—Your "righteousness and peace and joy in the Holy Spirit" (Romans 14:17)—as it is in heaven. Imagine heaven raining down righteousness, peace and joy in me, flowing out as a well of living water. I was called out in a service a couple of weeks ago, and the pastor told me that I would lead the people into joy.… I want my heart to be an open door, a portal to receive from heaven's throne. All the promises, all the blessings, the inheritance that belongs to me because of the blood of Jesus Christ, the finished work at Calvary—I want it all now! I don't want to squander and misuse like the prodigal son, but live the abundant life that God predestined for me, fulfilling my purpose and reaching my destiny.… Here I am, Lord. Mold me and make me; use me for Your glory; manifest Your will through me. It is through You that I live and move and have my being (Acts 17:28). Flow through me, Holy Spirit. Be not stagnant and still; stir up the fallow ground in me so that Your rain saturates me and waters the seeds that You have sown in me. May deep roots take hold in my soul and grow like a tree planted by the rivers of living water (Psalm 1:3). Produce the fruits of Your Spirit so that all may partake and be filled. Nourish and flourish in me, Lord, so the weeds of doubt may be choked and the symptoms that I feel may blow away like the white petals of a dandelion in the summer air. I am ready, Lord. Hear my call. I AM READY, LORD, RIGHT NOW!

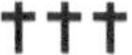

40

What's Next?

May 16, 2015 (Saturday)

MATTHEW 9:6-7 — *Then He said to the paralytic, "Arise, take up your bed, and go to your house." And he arose and departed to his house.*

✝✝✝

What an experience! Never have I been impacted through a daily devotional as I have with this forty-day journey. From day one, the Lord has shown Himself to me in real and tangible ways: touching my body, downloading songs into my spirit-man, journaling with a resolve and conviction as the Spirit wrote to me and through me. With great expectation and anticipation, I eagerly waited for the next day's journey. As I look at my notes and journal pages, there is so much to digest. So much has been poured into me over the last forty-plus days; my belly is full, overflowing with rivers of living water. I came to the table hungry and thirsty and have feasted. Now I am full of more faith, full of more God. I have opened my heart and invited the Trinity in, and They have come in and supped with me (Revelation 3:20). My relationship with the Trinity has grown in volumes, and my desire is for more and more— more of the Spirit, more of His fruit, more of His living waters flowing up and out of my soul. This is just the beginning on my journey to be whole. Whatever He says, whatever it takes, I will do. My destiny is in His hands; my determination and desire are true. My destination is the realm of Divine Health and Wholeness, entering through faith's portal door. I am on my way, closer than I've ever been. I thank You, Lord, for the journey's commencement. Looking forward to graduation's end. Still on my journey.

✝✝✝

These forty-plus days have been amazing! My relationship with the Trinity has grown deeper and more intimate than it has ever been. I have spent more time in the Word than I ever have. My time in prayer and communication with the Lord has been fluid; and inwardly I feel closer and more connected to the Spirit that resides and abides within. I can say with truth that I really love the Lord because I am in a relationship with Him. I know I faltered and did not put Him first, and consequently the forty days took much longer to complete than anticipated. I am sorry and have asked forgiveness and don't believe that God is holding that against me, for He has continued to bless me and give me His wisdom through my journaling. This is not an ending but a beginning; and I anticipate many more forty-day journeys in the future. I feel different in my being—more spirit than body. My spirit-man is resurrected and alive; and I am beginning to feel whole! I will continue this lifestyle until Jesus comes! Thank you, Trinity, for such an amazing journey!

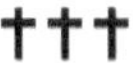

Afterwords

THE LORD, Who is the fountain of wisdom, wants to teach us; and often He speaks through one of His servants—like the sermon of a preacher, the song of a singer, the dance of a dancer. At other times the lessons are of such value that He uses the *lifetime* of one whom He has chosen. Such is the life of Joy Marlena Lambe. Such is the richness of *Finding Joy*.

Through her search for God, for healing, for wholeness, Joy found all. I believe Joy also found one of the deepest secrets of life, the security of knowing oneself enough to give oneself unreservedly to others. That is what Joy did in her sojourn here on earth. That is who Joy was to all of us. That is what Joy left us in the pages of her journal.

Joy was my friend and sister. I loved her dearly. She was compassionate, sensitive, knowing and able to smile and laugh at life's many varied moments. *Finding Joy* is, in many ways, her kind but sincere directive to us to be sure to find joy along this road of life. It is salve for the soul, poured from the heart of one who found her peace, her Joy, her secret place in the Lord—and who desired that we find ours too.

Dr. Vanessa Wynder Quainoo
Harrington School of Communication and Media
University of Rhode Island

WHILE READING JOY'S JOURNAL, the song "Through It All" by Andréa Crouch rang through my mind. I thought, *This song is the essence of Joy's learning to trust God through her health issues to her state of complete peace.* I was touched and inspired seeing Joy, in the midst of her illness, apply to her life the Word she studied, resulting in growth, healing and peace in her mind, body and soul.

As I witnessed Joy go through various bouts with cancer, including visits to the emergency room, some of which led to admission, I also witnessed her spiritual growth as God strengthened her determination to stay positive and believe His Word. I saw the Lord touch her body time after time and return her to some degree of regular functioning.

I saw Joy continually push through her sickness and pain to faithfully attend worship services, provide weekly tutoring sessions for community children and youth, and freely share her creative abilities among the church auxiliaries as they ministered within and beyond the church family. Now I see how she took the steps to get through each day. It was because of the strength she had built during this forty-day journey and her growing connection to the Trinity—God the Father, God the Son and God the Holy Spirit.

Joy was like a daughter to me, and our family loved her dearly. I thank God for her—and the love she had for God, her family, her Over the Top sisters, her music and the saints. She was a talented and dedicated woman who was a champion for educating our youth. She will be with us forever as we remember her creativity in the plays she wrote and directed, her artistry as we planned for annual programs and decorated for special events, her generosity as we fellowshipped with good food, and her competitiveness when we played her favorite games. Her spirit of excellence remains part of the fiber of the groups she participated in.

Joy left here testifying to others of the goodness of God and what He requires of us. I thank God for her life.

Elaine J. Gamble
Church of God in Christ for All Saints

IN THE EARLY MORNING HOURS of Saturday, February 23, 2019, I had a dream that brought a degree of comfort and closure while remembering an arduous yet beautiful life. The site of the dream was our family home on Carlton Street in Morristown, New Jersey, which Joy called home the first three and the final thirty years of her human sojourn.

✝✝✝

I am standing in the kitchen near the water dispenser talking with someone. A small person with the body of a child and the face of an adult walks past us. I recognize the face as Joy and am totally surprised how freely she moves past us. No hint of past infirmity. She is dressed in black, with a full Afro. She doesn't speak as she walks through the kitchen and takes her place at the dining room table, where she often worked and ate....

As I sit on the sofa in the living room, an adult, a younger version of Joy's mother without infirmity, walks up the stairs to the second floor. Joy, now a toddler in a bright print dress, too small to take hold of the handrail and walk upright, follows behind crawling up the stairs. Beautiful image of mother and child....

I go upstairs and enter the bedroom to the right at the top of the stairs. In the room is Joy's mother talking with an adult male, whom I cannot identify. Joy, now an infant, is wrapped in a blanket lying on the bed against the wall to the right. She is completely covered, with only her head and face in view. Again a mix of young and old, with a short Afro and wide brown eyes wise from her journey. I approach Joy, place my hand on her, and say, "You are beautiful." For a moment we look at each other. She closes her eyes. The dream ends.

✝✝✝

Later I realize that this last image of Joy mirrors my first sight of her when, in February 1965, I held her briefly after she and her mother arrived at the airport coming from Bermuda. Now as I remember Joy, this innocent yet wise infant comes into view, displacing the image of her final moments in human form. A reminder of the bountiful mysteries of life, as the Apostle Paul writes:

> *We know in part and we prophesy in part. But when that which is perfect has come, then that which is in part will be done away....For now we see in a mirror, dimly, but then face to face. Now I know in part, but then I shall know just as I also am known* (1 Corinthians 13:9-10, 12).

Sacred Journey...from beginning to end, from *Beginning* to *Beginning*.

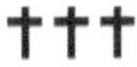

O little one
child of the mourning
firstborn
first gone
> how we miss you
> how we miss you

O little one
gem of creation
formed with such promise
now gone forever
> how we mourn you
> how we mourn you

O little one
warm ray of sunshine
breaking through the clouds
but just for a moment
> how we loved you
> how we loved you

O little one
gentle fragrant flower
blooming for a season
now returning to our Mother
> we hold you
> we release you

John Anthony Rogers
"Uncle John"

AS I READ *Finding Joy*, I was overwhelmed by the manifestation of healing that my sister ultimately experienced. Though cancer was a physical giant in Joy's life, like many of us she had other internal giants waging war against her soul, purpose, creativity, and peace.

As a gifted musician, talented play writer, educator, smart, insightful, caring, and the list goes on, my sister had creativity bursting at the seams. But life has a way of challenging our God-given greatness despite our being created in the image and likeness of God. If we are not careful, the enemy will cause us to forget how amazing we are and the priceless value that we carry.

Jesus says the thief comes to steal, kill, and ultimately destroy but that He has come that we might have life more abundantly (John 10:10). Thieves come after those things that have great value; and our value is not in what we do but in who we are! So when Joy's diagnosis came, my primary concern was not the cancer but the healing of her soul.

Jesus asks the question, What does it profit to gain the whole world and lose your soul? (Mark 8:36-37). I believe your soul is your mind, your will, and your emotions; and when these begin to heal, it positively affects how you see yourself and empowers you to be, not just to do. The challenge with long-term sickness or trauma is that it tends to become and overtake your true identity. You are not your sickness or trauma. You are greater than these, and the fight is to see beyond what you are going through. It's not an easy process, but it is necessary.

I saw Joy wrestling with the "why" of her condition while also struggling to embrace, or to be embraced by, the grace of God's unmerited favor. But there is nothing we can do to deserve the love, goodness, peace and favor of God. We just have to receive it. The challenge for many of us is having grown up in environments where love had strings attached or prerequisites to qualify for it. That was the fight—the fight for worth in order to receive what already is our God-given right to possess.

During Joy's seventeen-year journey, I saw her fight this fight for life; but I also saw life respond and begin to emerge from her, life that was more than just existing but living. I saw her creativity begin to soar again and purpose rise within. She began to live, but it was an everyday fight. So my prayer for my sister is now my prayer for you: a desire that your relationship with God and finding peace will become a realized priority in your life. You are worthy of love; receive it.

As I think about *Finding Joy*, this project is the answer to prayer that I have longed for. Joy literally went from running from God to running to Him and falling back in love with her Savior, discovering her purpose, and ministering profound revelation to those that are sick and hurting. For the seventeen years my sister battled cancer, she fought beyond the disease and found the God of her salvation; and through that relationship, she found peace and now is helping others to do the same. She has won the good fight of faith!

Rev. Jonathan E. Lambe
Chief Executive Officer, REIGN LIFE

We thank You, God, for the gift of Joy.

Thank You for loaning us another of Your treasures, allowing us to see and experience Your kindness and generosity and faithfulness manifest in and through her.

Thank You for Presence throughout her journey; for Spirit calling, guiding, comforting, encouraging on the path of Divine Health and Wholeness.

Thank You for all those sent to care, embrace, admonish, encourage, nurture and comfort.

Thank You for eternal love, peace and rest.

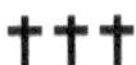

Romans 8:26-28, NIV

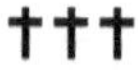

About the Author

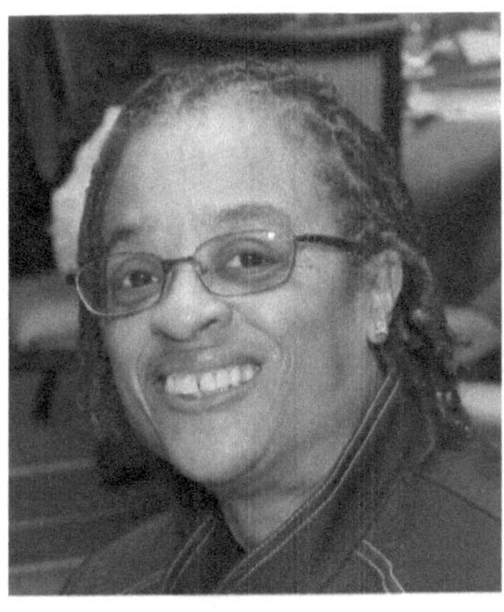

Joy Marlena Lambe was born on Sunday, December 13, 1964, into an African American family rooted in Holiness-Pentecostal traditions. Her parents and grandparents were leaders of religious congregations, which became her primary nurturing communities. In her teens, Joy transitioned from the local public school in Ashaway, RI, to The Williams School in New London, CT, a private day school several miles from her home community. After graduating high school, she spent four years at Wesleyan University in Middletown, CT, majoring in music. Exposed to new cultures and experiences, Joy had a season of exploration as she sought to determine her own values. After graduating college, she eventually returned to the home of her grandparents, where she had spent her first three years of life. Soon she reconnected with the faith community of her earliest years, and the journey of embracing and being embraced by that community ensued. This was the context for Joy's sojourn with cancer and her manifesting the loving presence of Christ until her passing on Thursday, May 3, 2018.

www.ingramcontent.com/pod-product-compliance
Lightning Source LLC
Chambersburg PA
CBHW031135250726
48655CB00002B/686